GOUT

FOOD

LIST

TABLE OF CONTENT

LOW-SODIUM BROTH

HERBS AND SPICES

OLIVE OIL

GREEN TEA

WATER

LOW-FAT CHEESE

VINEGAR

LOW-FAT DAIRY

Low-fat or non-fat milk, yogurt, and cheese can help reduce gout symptoms.

For individuals grappling with the painful and often debilitating condition of gout, the journey toward effective management can be both challenging and complex. Gout, characterized by the sudden and severe inflammation of joints due to the accumulation of uric acid crystals, demands careful attention to dietary choices. Amidst the myriad of considerations, one nutritional ally stands out – low-fat dairy.

Benefits of Low-Fat Dairy for Gout Patients:

1. Reduced Uric Acid Levels: Low-fat dairy products, such as milk, yogurt, and cheese, have been linked to a decrease in uric acid levels. These products are rich in a specific protein known as casein, which appears to have a protective effect against gout by aiding in the excretion of uric acid.

2. Calcium and Vitamin D: Low-fat dairy is a fantastic source of calcium and vitamin D. These nutrients are crucial for maintaining strong bones and overall health, particularly for individuals who may be taking medications for gout that can affect bone health.

3. Protein Source: Dairy products offer a source of high-quality protein without the purine content found in some meat and seafood, which can trigger gout attacks. Incorporating low-fat dairy can help gout patients meet their protein needs without exacerbating their condition.

4. Weight Management: Obesity is a risk factor for gout, and maintaining a healthy weight is essential for gout management. Low-fat dairy products provide essential nutrients while being lower in calories and unhealthy saturated fats, supporting weight control efforts.

5. Gut Health: Emerging research suggests that the probiotics found in yogurt may have a positive

impact on gut health, potentially reducing inflammation, which is a key factor in gout.

6. Satiety and Portion Control: Low-fat dairy can help gout patients feel satisfied, potentially reducing the consumption of high-purine foods, sweets, and processed snacks that can contribute to gout flares.

Incorporating low-fat dairy into a gout-friendly diet can be a smart and nutritious choice. However, individual responses to dietary changes may vary, so it's essential for gout patients to work closely with healthcare providers or registered dietitians to create a personalized nutrition plan that suits their specific needs and triggers.

WHOLE GRAINS

Foods like whole wheat bread, brown rice, and oatmeal provide essential nutrients and fiber.

For individuals living with gout, dietary choices play a pivotal role in managing this painful condition effectively. Among the many dietary options available, whole grains stand out as a valuable ally in the battle against gout. Whole grains encompass a diverse group of nutritious foods such as brown rice, quinoa, whole wheat, oats, and barley, each of which offers a host of benefits to those seeking to alleviate gout symptoms and reduce the risk of flare-ups.

BENEFITS OF WHOLE GRAINS FOR GOUT PATIENTS:

1. Low in Purines: Whole grains are naturally low in purines, the compounds that break down into uric acid, the culprit behind gout. By incorporating whole grains into your diet, you minimize the intake of purines, helping to keep uric acid levels in check.

2. Rich in Fiber: Whole grains are an excellent source of dietary fiber, which aids in maintaining a healthy weight, an essential aspect of gout management. Fiber also assists in reducing insulin resistance, potentially lowering uric acid levels.

3. Anti-Inflammatory Properties: Whole grains contain antioxidants and anti-inflammatory compounds that can help reduce inflammation in the body, easing the discomfort associated with gout attacks.

4. Stabilizes Blood Sugar: Whole grains have a low glycemic index, which means they release sugar into the bloodstream slowly, preventing rapid spikes in blood sugar levels. This stable blood sugar control is particularly important for gout patients, as diabetes is a common comorbidity.

5. Heart Health: Gout patients often have an increased risk of cardiovascular problems. Whole grains contribute to heart health by promoting

lower cholesterol levels and reducing the risk of heart disease.

6. Satiety: Whole grains provide a sense of fullness and satisfaction, reducing the temptation to consume high-purine, high-calorie foods that can exacerbate gout symptoms.

VEGETABLES

Adding a variety of non-cruciferous veggies like kale, spinach, and bell peppers into your diet.

For individuals grappling with gout, the inclusion of vegetables in their diet offers a remarkable opportunity for relief and overall improved well-being. These vibrant and nutrient-packed plant foods not only tantalize the palate but also serve as potent allies in the battle against gout's painful symptoms. Vegetables are naturally low in purines, compounds that break down into uric acid and contribute to gout flares, making them an essential component of a gout-friendly diet. Rich in essential vitamins, minerals, and dietary fiber, vegetables aid in maintaining a healthy weight and promoting proper digestion, both of which are vital in managing gout. Moreover, the antioxidants found abundantly in vegetables can help reduce inflammation and lower uric acid levels, providing much-needed relief from the discomfort associated with gout. By embracing a diet replete with a rainbow of vegetables, gout patients can savor not only the delicious flavors but also the myriad benefits these nutrient-dense foods offer, paving the way to a healthier, more comfortable life.

LEGUMES

lentils, chickpeas, and tofu are excellent sources of protein without the high purine content of meats.

Legumes, a diverse family of nutrient-rich plant foods, hold a special place in the diets of gout patients due to their remarkable benefits. These leguminous wonders, which encompass beans, lentils, chickpeas, and peas, offer a powerful combination of nutrition and gout management. For those grappling with the discomfort of gout, legumes present a culinary ally that not only tantalizes the taste buds but also promotes joint health. Legumes are celebrated for their low purine content, a crucial factor in gout management as purines break down into uric acid, a primary culprit behind gout flare-ups. Their high fiber content aids in weight management, a key aspect of gout control, by helping individuals maintain a healthy weight or lose excess pounds. Additionally, legumes are brimming with essential nutrients like potassium, which may counteract the harmful effects of uric acid, and antioxidants that combat inflammation, providing relief to gout-afflicted joints. Including legumes into a gout-conscious diet not only enhances overall nutrition but also contributes to the prevention and management of gout, granting patients a flavorful and nutritious path toward improved joint health.

NUTS

Almonds, walnuts, and flaxseeds can be part of a gout-friendly diet in moderation.

Nuts, nature's little powerhouses of nutrition, offer a wealth of benefits to gout patients, making them a valuable addition to a gout-friendly diet. Rich in heart-healthy unsaturated fats, nuts not only provide satiety but also help maintain a healthy body weight, a crucial factor in managing gout. Furthermore, these crunchy treats boast low purine content, reducing the risk of uric acid buildup that can trigger painful gout attacks. Additionally, nuts are packed with essential nutrients, including fiber, antioxidants, and anti-inflammatory compounds, which collectively contribute to reducing inflammation and alleviating gout symptoms. By incorporating a variety of nuts like almonds, walnuts, and pistachios into their diet, gout patients can enjoy a convenient and nutritious snack option that not only satisfies cravings but also supports their overall health and well-being. So, whether sprinkled on salads, blended into smoothies, or simply enjoyed by the handful, nuts can be a delicious and gout-friendly addition to a balanced diet, helping individuals with gout take proactive steps towards managing their condition and achieving better overall health.

LEAN PROTEINS

Choose skinless poultry, lean cuts of beef or pork, and fish (except high-purine varieties like sardines and anchovies).

 Lean proteins, such as skinless poultry, fish, and select cuts of lean meats, not only satisfy the palate but also hold the key to mitigating the symptoms and frequency of gout attacks. These protein sources are distinguished by their lower purine content, a crucial consideration for those with gout, as high purine levels can contribute to the accumulation of uric acid crystals in the joints, leading to painful inflammation and discomfort. Lean proteins offer a multifaceted array of benefits to gout patients, ranging from aiding in the reduction of uric acid levels to promoting overall joint health. Their significance extends beyond mere sustenance, encompassing a realm of therapeutic advantages that elevate them to a fundamental component of a gout-friendly diet.

1. Purine Moderation: Lean proteins are naturally low in purines, which are chemical compounds that break down into uric acid in the body. By consuming lean proteins, gout patients can better

manage their purine intake, reducing the likelihood of elevated uric acid levels and subsequent gout flares.

2. Uric Acid Regulation: Lean proteins can aid in the regulation of uric acid production and excretion, thus helping to maintain healthy uric acid levels in the bloodstream. This critical balance is essential for preventing the formation of uric acid crystals that trigger gout attacks.

3. Weight Management: Obesity and excess body weight are known risk factors for gout. Lean proteins are not only lower in fat but also provide satiety, helping gout patients maintain a healthy weight or achieve weight loss goals, reducing the strain on joints and the likelihood of gout episodes.

4. Joint Health: Adequate protein intake is crucial for maintaining and repairing joint tissues. Lean proteins provide essential amino acids and nutrients that support overall joint health, potentially mitigating the severity of gout-related joint pain and inflammation.

5. Muscle Preservation: Gout patients are often encouraged to stay active, as regular exercise can help manage the condition. Lean proteins play a pivotal role in muscle preservation, ensuring that individuals with gout can engage in physical activities without compromising muscle mass.

6. Heart Health: Gout is often associated with other cardiovascular risk factors. Lean proteins, particularly fish, are rich in heart-healthy omega-3 fatty acids, which can help improve cardiovascular health and reduce the risk of associated conditions.

EGGS

Eggs are a good source of protein and can be included in your diet.

Eggs, often referred to as nature's nutritional powerhouse, offer a multitude of benefits to individuals grappling with gout, a form of arthritis caused by the buildup of uric acid crystals in the joints. Rich in high-quality protein, eggs provide gout patients with a valuable source of essential amino acids while offering a low-purine alternative to certain high-purine animal proteins that can exacerbate gout symptoms. Furthermore, eggs are renowned for their choline content, a vital nutrient that aids in reducing inflammation and supporting liver function crucial for those with gout, as the liver plays a pivotal role in uric acid regulation. The presence of vitamin D in eggs is an additional boon, as it aids in calcium absorption and bone health, which is particularly significant for gout sufferers who may experience joint damage over time. Lastly, eggs are a versatile culinary ingredient, allowing gout patients to savor a variety of enjoyable and gout-friendly dishes, from protein-packed omelets to nutrient-rich salads, all while managing their condition and savoring the goodness of a well-rounded diet.

WHOLE-GRAIN PASTA

Opt for whole-grain pasta instead of refined white pasta.

Whole-grain pasta offers a tantalizing and health-conscious alternative for individuals grappling with Unlike traditional refined pasta, whole-grain pasta is a nutritional powerhouse, brimming with benefits tailored to alleviate the challenges of gout. Packed with essential nutrients, including fiber, vitamins, and minerals, it plays a pivotal role in maintaining a well-rounded diet while minimizing the risk of gout flare-ups. Its high fiber content facilitates improved digestion and promotes a gradual release of carbohydrates, thereby preventing rapid spikes in blood sugar levels—an important consideration for individuals with gout, as high blood sugar may exacerbate the condition. Furthermore, the presence of antioxidants in whole-grain pasta combats inflammation, a key factor in gout's painful symptoms. Additionally, the relatively low purine content in whole grains, compared to certain animal-based proteins, aids in reducing uric acid production—a pivotal aspect of gout management. As if these advantages weren't compelling enough, whole-grain pasta's delectable taste and versatility make it a delightful addition to a gout-friendly menu, ensuring that individuals with gout can savor the pleasure of pasta while safeguarding their joint health.

QUINOA

This ancient grain is high in protein and can be a good alternative to rice.

Quinoa, often referred to as the "superfood of the Andes," is a versatile and nutritious grain-like seed that has gained worldwide popularity for its remarkable health benefits. While it is celebrated for its positive impact on various aspects of well-being, its significance extends to those grappling with gout—a painful form of arthritis caused by the buildup of uric acid crystals in the joints. In this discussion, we delve into the exceptional advantages that quinoa offers to individuals managing gout, highlighting how this nutrient-packed grain can be a valuable addition to their dietary arsenal.

Benefits of Quinoa for Gout Patients:

Gout patients can find solace in the numerous advantages that quinoa brings to their dietary choices. Firstly, quinoa is low in purines, which are compounds that break down into uric acid. This makes it a gout-friendly source of plant-based protein, allowing individuals to meet their protein needs without exacerbating uric acid levels. Furthermore, quinoa is rich in fiber, which supports overall digestive health and may help regulate weight—a crucial factor in gout management. Its impressive nutrient profile also includes essential vitamins and minerals like magnesium, which is believed to help reduce the frequency and severity of gout attacks. Additionally, quinoa's anti-inflammatory properties can aid in alleviating the pain and discomfort associated with gout, contributing to improved joint health and overall quality of life. Moreover, its versatility in the kitchen allows gout patients to savor a wide range of delectable dishes, providing a delightful and nourishing culinary experience. Whether enjoyed in salads, as a side dish, or as a protein-rich main course, quinoa offers gout patients a flavorful and nutritious alternative that aligns with their dietary needs and aids in the management of this challenging condition.

TOFU

A low-purine source of plant-based protein.

Tofu, the versatile plant-based protein that can be a game-changer for individuals managing gout. Tofu, derived from soybeans, offers a plethora of benefits uniquely suited to the dietary needs of gout patients. This nutrient-packed food is renowned for its low-purine content, making it a safe and delicious addition to gout-friendly diets. Tofu is not only a rich source of high-quality protein, aiding in muscle maintenance and repair, but it also provides essential minerals like calcium and magnesium, which contribute to bone health. Furthermore, tofu is a heart-healthy choice, as it contains minimal saturated fat and no cholesterol, reducing the risk of cardiovascular complications often associated with gout. Its natural soy compounds, including isoflavones, may even possess anti-inflammatory properties, potentially offering relief from gout-related pain and swelling. Tofu's culinary adaptability allows for a wide range of savory and sweet preparations, ensuring that gout patients can savor satisfying meals without compromising on taste, all while reaping the benefits of this remarkable, gout-friendly superfood.

BEANS

Kidney beans, black beans, and navy beans are low in purines.

For individuals battling the discomfort and pain of gout, incorporating beans into their diet can be a welcome and nutritious addition. Beans, a staple in many cuisines around the world, offer a multitude of benefits to gout patients. These legumes, which include varieties such as kidney beans, black beans, and lentils, are not only a source of plant-based protein but also rich in fiber and essential nutrients. Gout, a form of arthritis, results from the accumulation of uric acid crystals in the joints, often causing severe pain and inflammation. Beans, by nature, are low in purines, compounds that metabolize into uric acid in the body. This makes them a gout-friendly choice as they are less likely to trigger gout attacks or worsen existing symptoms. Additionally, the high fiber content in beans aids in maintaining a healthy weight, which is crucial for gout management, as excess body weight is a known risk factor for the condition. Furthermore, beans promote better blood sugar control, a vital consideration for those with gout as diabetes is often a comorbidity. Their versatility in various recipes allows gout patients to enjoy flavorful and satisfying meals while actively supporting their joint health. With their combination of low purine content, fiber, and essential nutrients, beans emerge as a valuable dietary ally for gout patients, offering not only relief from painful symptoms but also contributing to an overall healthier lifestyle.

MUSHROOMS

Most mushrooms are considered low-purine and can be enjoyed in moderation.

Mushrooms, often regarded as culinary marvels, offer a tantalizing world of flavors and textures to gout patients while providing a host of health benefits. Gout can be managed effectively through dietary choices. Incorporating mushrooms into the diet presents an exciting opportunity for gout patients. These earthy gems are naturally low in purines, the compounds that break down into uric acid, making them an excellent addition to gout-friendly menus. Beyond their purine content, mushrooms boast numerous advantages for gout sufferers. They are a rich source of dietary fiber, aiding in digestion and weight management, a crucial aspect of gout control. Additionally, mushrooms contain bioactive compounds such as beta-glucans, which have anti-inflammatory properties that may help alleviate gout-related joint pain and inflammation. Furthermore, mushrooms are packed with essential nutrients, including vitamins, minerals, and antioxidants, which support overall health and strengthen the immune system. As versatile ingredients that can be incorporated into various dishes, mushrooms not only enhance the culinary experience for gout patients but also contribute to a well-rounded, uric acid-conscious diet that promotes both symptom relief and long-term wellness.

OATS

Oatmeal and oats are heart-healthy and suitable for a gout diet.

Oats, often hailed as a nutritional powerhouse, offer a myriad of health benefits, and for individuals battling gout, they emerge as a particularly promising dietary ally. Managing gout necessitates a comprehensive approach, and the inclusion of oats in the diet is a wise choice. These unassuming grains are a rich source of essential nutrients and possess unique properties that can be instrumental in mitigating the symptoms and reducing the risk of gout attacks. In this discussion, we delve into the remarkable benefits of oats for gout patients, shedding light on how this versatile food can be an integral part of a gout-friendly diet.

Benefits of Oats for Gout Patients:

Oats provide several key advantages for individuals grappling with gout:

1. Low in Purines: Oats are naturally low in purines, compounds that break down into uric acid. A diet

low in purines can help prevent the buildup of uric acid crystals in the joints, reducing the frequency and severity of gout attacks.

2. Rich in Fiber: Oats are a superb source of soluble fiber, which can aid in weight management and lower the risk of obesity—a significant risk factor for gout. Additionally, fiber promotes better digestion and helps regulate blood sugar levels, potentially reducing insulin resistance, which is often associated with gout.

3. Anti-Inflammatory Properties: Oats contain antioxidants and anti-inflammatory compounds that may help soothe gout-related joint inflammation and discomfort.

4. Heart Health: Gout and heart disease often coexist. Oats' cholesterol-lowering properties can benefit gout patients by promoting overall cardiovascular health, an essential aspect of gout management.

5. Satiety and Weight Control: Oats' ability to keep you feeling full can support weight control efforts, preventing excessive weight gain that can exacerbate gout symptoms.

Incorporating oats into a gout-conscious diet can be a delicious and nutritious strategy for managing this challenging condition. Whether enjoyed as a warm bowl of oatmeal, added to smoothies, or used as a base for savory dishes, oats offer a versatile and satisfying way to support gout management and promote overall well-being.

BROWN RICE

A healthier choice compared to white rice.

Including brown rice as a dietary staple offers a wealth of benefits to individuals managing gout, a condition characterized by the accumulation of uric acid crystals in the joints. Brown rice stands out as a nutritional powerhouse in the quest for better gout management, thanks to its unique composition and numerous advantages. Unlike refined white rice, brown rice retains its outer bran layer and germ, which harbor essential nutrients, fiber, and compounds beneficial to gout patients. Its high fiber content aids in stabilizing blood sugar levels, reducing insulin spikes, and supporting overall metabolic health—crucial factors for individuals with gout who are often at risk of developing metabolic disorders. Furthermore, brown rice boasts a lower glycemic index (GI) compared to white rice, meaning it is digested more slowly, helping to prevent rapid increases in blood sugar. This slow digestion also promotes a feeling of fullness, potentially aiding in weight management a key component of gout control. Brown rice is a reliable source of essential B vitamins, such as niacin and B6, which play a role in lowering uric acid levels in the body, thus offering a natural defense against gout flares. The magnesium content in brown rice is another valuable asset, as it helps regulate blood pressure and may indirectly contribute to gout management by reducing the risk of hypertension, a condition commonly associated with gout. In sum, incorporating brown rice into a gout-friendly diet not only enhances nutritional intake but also assists in stabilizing blood sugar, managing weight, and potentially mitigating the risk of gout flares making it a valuable ally for those on the journey to gout relief and overall well-being.

BARLEY

Another whole grain that can be incorporated into various dishes.

Barley, a humble grain often overlooked in modern diets, emerges as a nutritional gem for individuals grappling with gout a form of arthritis characterized by painful joint inflammation triggered by elevated uric acid levels. As we delve into the world of barley, we discover a versatile and wholesome ingredient that not only tantalizes the taste buds but also offers a host of benefits to those managing gout. Rich in dietary fiber, barley aids in regulating blood sugar levels and promoting a steady release of insulin, thereby reducing the risk of insulin resistance often associated with gout. Furthermore, this unassuming grain boasts a relatively low purine content compared to other protein sources, which can help mitigate the uric acid buildup responsible for gout attacks. Barley's high-fiber profile contributes to weight management, a crucial aspect of gout management, as excess weight can exacerbate gout symptoms. Its fiber content also aids in maintaining a healthy gut microbiome, potentially reducing inflammation—a primary concern for gout sufferers. Additionally, barley is replete with antioxidants, which can combat oxidative stress and inflammation in the body. Embracing barley as a dietary staple not only adds a layer of culinary delight to gout-friendly meals but also offers a valuable ally in the ongoing battle against gout, supporting overall health and well-being.

LOW-FAT YOGURT

A good source of protein and probiotics for gut health.

Low-fat yogurt as a dietary ally for individuals grappling with gout is a smart and flavorful choice that offers a multitude of benefits. Low-fat yogurt, a rich source of essential nutrients, including calcium, probiotics, and protein, can play a pivotal role in managing this condition. Its low purine content helps mitigate the risk of uric acid accumulation, reducing the likelihood of painful gout attacks. Moreover, the calcium in low-fat yogurt supports overall bone health and can counteract the potential bone-weakening effects of long-term gout medications. Additionally, the probiotics found in yogurt may contribute to improved gut health and a balanced gut microbiome, potentially aiding in reducing inflammation—a key factor in gout flare-ups. Furthermore, the protein content of low-fat yogurt provides a valuable energy source while helping to maintain muscle mass. As a versatile food, low-fat yogurt can be enjoyed in various ways, from smoothies and parfaits to savory dips and salad dressings, making it an accessible and delectable addition to a gout-friendly diet that supports overall well-being and helps keep gout symptoms at bay.

LOW-SODIUM BROTH

Use in cooking and soups to control sodium intake.

Low-sodium broth is typically made by simmering bones or vegetables in water and adding minimal salt or sodium. It can be prepared at home using bone-in meats, such as chicken, turkey, or beef, along with a medley of fresh vegetables and aromatic herbs. Alternatively, store-bought low-sodium broth options are readily available in most grocery stores, offering convenience to those with busy schedules.

Benefits of Low-Sodium Broth for Gout Patients:

1. Hydration: Adequate hydration is crucial for individuals with gout, as it helps flush excess uric acid from the body. Low-sodium broth is a flavorful way to increase daily fluid intake, keeping the joints lubricated and assisting in the removal of uric acid crystals.

2. Nutrient-Rich: Low-sodium broth is a source of essential nutrients like calcium, magnesium, and collagen. These nutrients play a role in joint health and may help alleviate gout symptoms by supporting overall joint function.

3. Flavor Enhancement: Gout-friendly diets often emphasize whole, unprocessed foods with reduced salt content. Low-sodium broth can be used to add depth and flavor to dishes without the excessive sodium that may exacerbate gout symptoms.

4. Weight Management: Gout is more common in individuals who are overweight or obese. Low-sodium broth can be part of a calorie-controlled, nutritious diet that aids in weight management, reducing the risk of gout flares.

5. Warmth and Comfort: Gout attacks can be particularly painful, and warm, soothing broths can provide comfort during flare-ups, promoting relaxation and well-being.

Adding low-sodium broth into your diet can be a flavorful and healthful choice for managing gout. It's essential, however, to continue consulting with a healthcare provider or registered dietitian for personalized dietary recommendations tailored to your specific condition and needs.

HERBS AND SPICES

Flavor dishes with herbs like basil, oregano, and rosemary instead of salt.

Gout often demands a multifaceted approach to management, and one element that holds immense promise in alleviating symptoms and reducing flare-ups is the inclusion of herbs and spices in the diet. These natural treasures have been used for centuries in various culinary traditions and medicinal practices, offering not only a burst of flavor but also a plethora of health benefits.

Preparation and Benefits of Herbs and Spices for Gout Patients:

1. Anti-Inflammatory Properties: Many herbs and spices possess potent anti-inflammatory properties, which can help reduce the swelling and discomfort associated with gout. Turmeric, for instance, contains curcumin, a powerful anti-

inflammatory compound known to alleviate joint pain.

2. Pain Relief: The warming properties of spices like ginger and cayenne pepper can provide natural pain relief to gout sufferers. These spices may help to ease the intensity of gout-related discomfort.

3. Improved Blood Circulation: Spices like cinnamon and cayenne pepper can aid in improving blood circulation, potentially assisting in the removal of uric acid crystals from the joints.

4. Antioxidant Rich: Many herbs and spices are packed with antioxidants, which can help combat oxidative stress and reduce the risk of inflammation. Basil, oregano, and thyme, for example, are rich in antioxidants that may support gout management.

5. Enhanced Flavor without Sodium: Gout patients are often advised to limit their sodium intake. Herbs and spices offer a flavorful alternative to

salt, allowing individuals to season their meals without increasing their sodium levels.

6. Natural Diuretics: Certain herbs like parsley and dandelion have natural diuretic properties that can promote the elimination of excess uric acid through urine.

7. Digestive Aid: Many spices aid digestion, which can be beneficial for individuals with gout. Ginger and peppermint, for instance, can help alleviate digestive discomfort.

8. Versatile Culinary Enhancement: Herbs and spices are incredibly versatile and can be incorporated into a wide range of dishes, making it easier for gout patients to enjoy flavorful meals while adhering to dietary restrictions.

As with any dietary changes, it's crucial for gout patients to consult with a healthcare provider or registered dietitian to ensure that herbs and spices are integrated into their diet safely and effectively.

When utilized thoughtfully, these natural ingredients can offer a flavorful and healthful addition to the gout management toolkit, providing not only relief from pain but also a path towards better overall well-being.

OLIVE OIL

Use olive oil in cooking and as a salad dressing.

Among the numerous dietary choices available, olive oil stands out as a remarkably beneficial and versatile option for gout patients. Not only does it lend exquisite flavor to a variety of dishes, but it also harbors a host of health advantages that can help individuals with gout lead a more comfortable and enjoyable life. In this discussion, we will explore the unique benefits of incorporating olive oil into the diet of gout patients and how it can contribute to their overall well-being.

Benefits of Olive Oil for Gout Patients:

1. Anti-Inflammatory Properties: Gout is fundamentally an inflammatory condition, and olive oil is renowned for its potent anti-inflammatory properties. The monounsaturated fats and antioxidants found in olive oil, particularly in extra virgin olive oil, can help reduce inflammation in the body, which is critical for managing gout symptoms.

2. Low in Purines: Gout is often exacerbated by the consumption of high-purine foods, as purines break down into uric acid, a key contributor to gout attacks. Olive oil is naturally low in purines, making it a safe and gout-friendly cooking oil.

3. Heart Health: Gout and cardiovascular health are closely linked. Olive oil promotes heart health by lowering bad cholesterol levels and reducing the risk of heart disease, a significant concern for gout patients who often have comorbid conditions. A healthy heart is vital for overall well-being.

4. Weight Management: Maintaining a healthy weight is crucial for gout management. Olive oil can be a valuable ally in weight control, as it can help you feel full and satisfied, reducing the temptation to overindulge in high-purine or unhealthy foods.

5. Joint Health: Gout primarily affects the joints, causing discomfort and pain. The anti-

inflammatory properties of olive oil can potentially alleviate some of this pain and improve joint mobility.

6. Versatility: Olive oil can be seamlessly integrated into a variety of dishes, from salads and sautés to dressings and marinades. Its versatility allows gout patients to enjoy a wide range of flavorful and satisfying meals while adhering to their dietary restrictions.

Incorporating olive oil into a gout-friendly diet can not only enhance the overall flavor of meals but also offer valuable health benefits that support gout management and improve quality of life for those living with this condition. However, it's essential to consume olive oil in moderation as part of a balanced diet tailored to individual needs and under the guidance of a healthcare provider or registered dietitian.

GREEN TEA

Known for its antioxidant properties, green tea can be a part of a gout-friendly diet.

Medications are often prescribed to manage gout, dietary choices can also play a crucial role in alleviating symptoms and preventing future flare-ups. One dietary option that has garnered increasing attention for its potential benefits in managing gout is green tea.

Benefits of Green Tea for Gout Patients:

1. Anti-Inflammatory Properties: Green tea is renowned for its anti-inflammatory properties, which can be particularly beneficial for individuals with gout. The inflammation associated with gout attacks is a major source of pain and discomfort, and green tea's compounds, particularly catechins, have been shown to reduce inflammation in various studies.

2. Uric Acid Regulation: Green tea may help regulate uric acid levels in the body. High uric acid

levels are a hallmark of gout, and by promoting the excretion of uric acid through the kidneys, green tea may assist in preventing the formation of uric acid crystals in the joints.

3. Antioxidant Effects: Green tea is rich in antioxidants, such as epigallocatechin gallate (EGCG), which can help protect the body's cells from oxidative damage. Gout is often associated with oxidative stress, and the antioxidant properties of green tea may help mitigate this stress, potentially reducing the severity and frequency of gout attacks.

4. Weight Management: Maintaining a healthy weight is essential for gout management, as excess body weight can increase the risk of gout and exacerbate symptoms. Green tea has been studied for its potential role in supporting weight loss and weight maintenance. By incorporating green tea into a healthy diet and lifestyle, gout patients may better manage their weight and reduce gout-related complications.

5. Hydration: Staying well-hydrated is crucial for gout patients to help flush excess uric acid from the body. Green tea, whether consumed hot or cold, contributes to daily fluid intake, aiding in hydration.

It's important to note that while green tea shows promise in aiding gout management, it should not be considered a standalone treatment. Incorporating green tea into a balanced diet can be a flavorful and potentially beneficial addition to a holistic approach to gout care.

WATER

Staying well-hydrated is essential for gout management.

Water is often hailed as the elixir of life, and its significance in maintaining good health cannot be overstated. For individuals grappling with gout, a type of arthritis caused by the buildup of uric acid crystals in the joints, the role of water takes on an even greater importance. Gout patients often experience painful joint inflammation and recurrent attacks, and proper hydration can be a valuable ally in managing this condition.

Benefits of Water for Gout Patients:

1. Uric Acid Dilution: One of the primary culprits in gout is elevated uric acid levels in the bloodstream. Drinking an ample amount of water helps dilute uric acid, making it easier for the kidneys to filter and excrete it from the body. This, in turn, reduces the risk of uric acid crystals forming in the joints.

2. Preventing Dehydration: Gout attacks can be triggered or exacerbated by dehydration. Insufficient water intake can lead to higher uric acid concentrations in the blood, potentially increasing the likelihood of painful flare-ups. Proper hydration helps maintain a balance in uric acid levels, reducing the risk of gout attacks.

3. Improved Joint Function: Well-hydrated joints are better lubricated, which can ease joint pain and discomfort associated with gout. Adequate water intake promotes better overall joint function and can help reduce the severity of symptoms during gout attacks.

4. Kidney Function: Gout is often associated with kidney health. Staying hydrated supports optimal kidney function, allowing these vital organs to efficiently process and excrete uric acid from the body. This can contribute to long-term management and prevention of gout-related complications.

5. Alleviating Pain: Gout attacks can be excruciatingly painful. While water alone cannot eliminate the pain, it can contribute to overall better health, potentially reducing the frequency and severity of gout episodes, leading to a better quality of life for gout patients.

Water is an essential and often overlooked component of managing gout. Proper hydration aids in diluting uric acid, preventing dehydration-triggered gout attacks, improving joint function, supporting kidney health, and alleviating pain. Gout patients should prioritize staying well-hydrated as part of their overall strategy for managing this condition effectively.

LOW-FAT CHEESE

Choose reduced-fat cheese options for a lower-purine source of dairy.

One dietary consideration that can positively impact gout management is the incorporation of low-fat cheese into your meal plan. Low-fat cheese is not only a delectable addition to your culinary repertoire but also offers several benefits for gout patients.

Benefits of Low-Fat Cheese for Gout Patients:

1. Reduced Purine Content: Gout patients are advised to limit their intake of purine-rich foods, as purines can contribute to elevated uric acid levels. Low-fat cheese, compared to full-fat versions, generally contains fewer purines, making it a safer choice for gout sufferers.

2. Moderate Protein Source: Low-fat cheese provides a moderate amount of protein, which is essential for tissue repair and overall health. It can

serve as a satisfying protein source without
overloading your system with excessive purines.

3. Calcium Richness: Dairy products like low-fat
cheese are rich in calcium, a mineral that may help
reduce the risk of gout attacks. Adequate calcium
intake may facilitate uric acid excretion and
support bone health.

4. Weight Management: Gout is often associated
with obesity. Choosing low-fat cheese as part of a
balanced diet can assist in weight management,
potentially reducing the frequency and severity of
gout flares.

5. Versatile Culinary Ingredient: Low-fat cheese is
incredibly versatile and can enhance the flavors of
a wide range of dishes. Whether incorporated into
salads, sandwiches, omelets, or enjoyed as a snack,
it can make adhering to a gout-friendly diet more
enjoyable.

Including low-fat cheese into your gout management plan can be a delicious and practical way to navigate dietary restrictions while promoting overall well-being. However, it's essential to consume it in moderation and as part of a balanced diet. Always consult with a healthcare professional or registered dietitian for personalized dietary recommendations tailored to your specific condition and needs.

VINEGAR

Some studies suggest that vinegar, particularly apple cider vinegar, may have potential gout benefits. Use it as a salad dressing or incorporate it into recipes.

Vinegar, a pantry staple known for its culinary versatility, has also gained recognition for its potential benefits in managing gout, a painful form of arthritis caused by the buildup of uric acid crystals in the joints. While gout management often involves medication and dietary adjustments, vinegar's natural properties have sparked interest among individuals seeking complementary ways to alleviate symptoms and support their overall health.

Benefits of Vinegar for Gout Patients:

1. Alkalizing Effect: Vinegar, particularly apple cider vinegar, is often considered alkaline in nature. An alkaline environment in the body may help neutralize excess uric acid, a key contributor to

gout attacks. By maintaining a more balanced pH level, vinegar may mitigate the risk of uric acid crystal formation.

2. Anti-Inflammatory Properties: Gout is characterized by painful inflammation in the joints. Vinegar's anti-inflammatory properties may offer relief by reducing swelling and discomfort in affected areas. Incorporating vinegar into your diet may aid in managing these painful flare-ups.

3. Weight Management: Obesity is a known risk factor for gout, as excess weight can lead to increased uric acid levels. Some studies suggest that vinegar may support weight management by promoting a feeling of fullness and reducing overall calorie intake. Maintaining a healthy weight can be instrumental in preventing gout attacks.

4. Blood Sugar Control: For individuals with both gout and diabetes, vinegar may play a dual role. It has been shown to improve insulin sensitivity and help regulate blood sugar levels. Stable blood sugar levels can contribute to better gout management.

5. Detoxification: Vinegar is believed to aid in detoxifying the body by assisting the liver and kidneys in processing waste products. Efficient detoxification processes can help reduce the load on these organs, potentially benefiting individuals with gout, as impaired kidney function can contribute to elevated uric acid levels.

While vinegar may offer several potential benefits for gout patients, it's crucial to approach its consumption with moderation. individual responses to dietary changes can vary. Integrating vinegar as part of a balanced diet and overall gout management strategy may help individuals find relief and improve their quality of life.

www.ingramcontent.com/pod-product-compliance
Lightning Source LLC
Chambersburg PA
CBHW070723260726
48660CB00007B/2702